THE FOUR MOST COMMON HAIRCUTS THAT ANYONE CAN MASTER

Utilize the efficient "connect the dot" diagrams and precision photographs throughout this book to:
Create the four most common haircuts, save hundreds of dollars each year, and enjoy quality time with your family and friends!

By Lisa MarieViggiano

THE FOUR MOST COMMON HAIRCUTS THAT ANYONE CAN MASTER

Utilize the efficient "connect the dot" diagrams and precision photographs throughout this book to:
Create the four most common haircuts, save hundreds of dollars each year and enjoy quality time with your family and friends!

Printed and Published in the USA 2005
First Printing
L & J Publishing and Graphics
P.O. Box 500868
Malabar, Florida 32950
Library of Congress Catalog Card Number: 2005936859
ISBN: 0-9770068-0-8

Introduction

Have you ever thought about the money you spend on haircuts in one year? What about the time wasted, waiting just to get into the chair; and as you go through the procedure of finally getting your hair cut?

In today's society, saving money is an issue if you are trying to raise a family. Most of us try to do anything we can to cut our expenses. In the United States, a haircut can cost from $8 to $25. If you have a family of four and you get your hair cut about once a month, your average expense could run around $816 a year. This money can be used wisely in many other areas. Time is also an issue in today's society. There never seems to be enough time. Most of us try to save time whenever we can so that we can spend it with our family and friends. Think about the time wasted going through the whole process of getting your hair cut. This time can be turned into quality time doing something more productive with your family and friends!

Dedication

For my husband John, who made it possible for me to fulfill my dream. He has given me all the support, encouragement and assurance needed throughout this long journey.

For my parents, who gave me direction throughout my life, and helped me to acquire my education that got me to where I am today.

For my friends Kendy and Kris who both supported me before during and after writing this book.

For Mark, Catie, Sarah and Justin, who participated in the photographs inside this book.

And finally, for all of my loyal clients throughout my career who helped me to stabilize my income, so that I could complete the goal of finishing this book.

Warning - Disclaimer!

All cosmetology tools are very sharp, and can cause serious bodily injuries to both children and adults. So, please handle them with care!
Neither the author nor publisher will be responsible for any accidental injury caused by any of the tools or explanations inside this book.
Cosmetology is considered a trade. A license in every state is required before it can be practiced as a business. Each state has individual requirements. If you are interested in studying this trade, research the information provided by your states Board of Cosmetology, or any cosmetology school in your area.
This book can be used as a guide for you and your family, for people currently attending cosmetology school, or for people planning to attend. Further education and a cosmetology license is required if you plan on cutting hair for income purposes.
You, the consumer are fully responsible for all of your own actions after purchasing this book.

Table of Contents

Chapter One
GETTING STARTED
The Four Simple Procedures and the Tools You Will Need

This book is going to show you several haircuts that you can easily do on your own. It contains all the simple steps and photographs needed for each cut. Each haircut is pretty basic; and will work well with straight, wavy, curly, fine or thick hair.

The four procedures needed to achieve these haircuts are as follows:

✂ *Procedure #1*: How to Cut the Bangs

✂ *Procedure #2:* How to Cut an All the Same Length Haircut

✂ *Procedure #3:* How to Cut Short Layers into the Hair

✂ *Procedure #4:* Cutting with Clippers

(See the following page for examples of each cut.)

Figure #1
(Procedure #1)

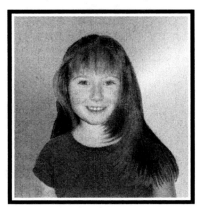

Figure #2
(Procedure #2)

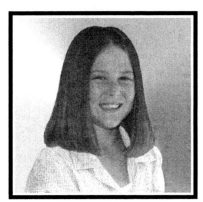

Figure #3
(Procedure #3)

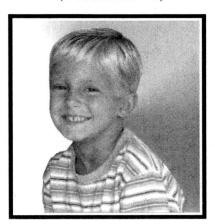

Figure#4
(Procedure #4)

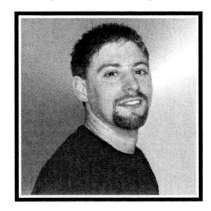

The only tools that you will need are:

✂ *An inexpensive pair of scissors*

✂ *An inexpensive pair of clippers*

✂ *A comb*

✂ *Four clips to hold the hair*

✂ *A cape or towel to cover the persons body from hair*

✂ *A water bottle*

You can purchase a pair of scissors and clippers together in a kit. You will find them sold this way at most supermarkets, pharmacies, and almost any retail store.

If you choose to purchase your clippers and scissors separately, there are many different brands to choose from. They can be purchased from any of the stores above.

Purchasing clippers and scissors from anywhere other than your local beauty supply store, might be the most affordable for you.

Although the scissors and clippers at your local beauty supplier may be more expensive, they are manufactured to last longer. The manufacturers keep in mind that these models will be used mostly by cosmetologists day after day. (See figures 5 and 6 on the following page).

Figure#5   **Figure#6**

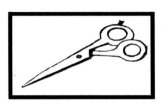   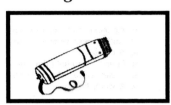

You can get by with any type of comb. The most efficient and longer lasting comb is made out of hard plastic. It is about 1 ¾ of an inch wide and 8 ¼ of an inch long. It can be purchased at your local beauty supply store. You may find something similar at a supermarket, pharmacy or retail store.

Once you get use to this larger comb, you will realize that it is much easier to comb through the hair because of its wider teeth. It will also allow you to work with more hair at one time. (See figure 7 below.)

Plastic clips can also be found at any of the stores above. (See figure 8 below.)

Figure#7   **Figure #8**

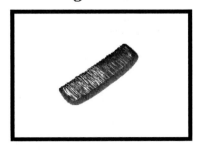   

If you wish to use a cape rather than a towel to cover the persons body from hair, this can be purchased at your local beauty supply store. (See figure #9 below.)

Figure #9

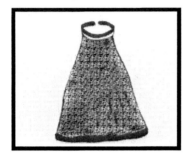

A water bottle can be purchased just about anywhere. (See figure #10 below.)

Figure #10

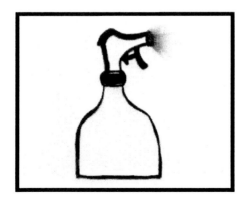

Before you begin, be sure to have a clean and organized work space. Place your tools in a safe area and make sure that they are easy to get to. This will make it much easier and less distracting for you.

Most importantly, have lots of fun!

Chapter Two
THINGS TO REMEMBER
The Secrets for a Successful Haircut

Here are a few secrets to guide you through the haircut. It is important that you consistently use this information throughout the book. You may have to refer back to this chapter several times.

✂ *Hair shrinks up when it dries.*

✂ *Hair shrinks up when it is curly or wavy.*

✂ *Hair shrinks up at any cowlick or growth pattern.*

✂ *To prevent cutting the hair too short, allow more room for the hair to shrink by leaving it a little longer where needed. (Although hair shrinks in several conditions, it is much easier to cut when it is wet with the exception of cutting the bangs.)*

✂ *Leave a little conditioner in the hair after shampooing it. This will make it easier to cut.*

✕ *If the hair contains any residue of heavy gels, hairsprays, or even chlorine and other minerals, it will be harder to cut. The finished cut could possibly turn out uneven. Before continuing the haircut, shampoo the hair with a "clarifying shampoo" to remove any residue.*

✕ *Hair is usually the thickest in density at the very back center of the head.*

✕ *Hair is usually medium in density on the sides of the head.*

✕ *Hair is usually the least dense around the very front of the head.*

✕ *When you are cutting, always make sure that you can see your guides. Visualize yourself "connecting the dots". Accomplish this in the most comfortable method to you. This book is simple to follow for both right and left-handed people.*

✕ *Pay special attention to your tool manuals so that you understand how to clean, disinfect, and oil your clippers and scissors. Take care of your tools regularly and you will get better results with your haircuts.*

Chapter Three
WHAT IS A HAIRLINE?
A Simple Procedure to Help You Locate the Hairline

The hairline is the area in which the hair grows out of around the neck, sides, above the ears, and the forehead. You can find the hairline by lifting the hair up in these specific areas around the head.

It is very important that you are familiar with the location of the hairline, because most people do not like their hair cut above it. Familiarizing yourself with this area will help you to achieve a more natural look when cutting the hair. (See figure 1 below.)

Figure#1

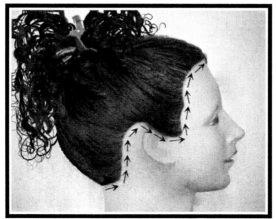

After finding the hairline, you can move on to chapter four. This chapter will show you an easy way to hold the scissors and comb together while cutting.

Keep in mind that Practice Makes Perfect!

Chapter Four
PRACTICE MAKES PERFECT
How to Hold the Scissors and Comb Together while cutting

When holding the scissors and comb together while cutting, you will consistantly be transferring the comb from one hand to the other. Before you start cutting, practice these simple steps with the help of the photographs provided on the following pages.

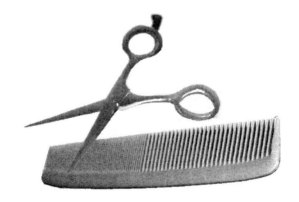

Step#1: Hold the scissors and comb together with the hand that has the most dexterity. If you are right handed, hold the scissors and comb with your right hand. If you are left handed, hold the scissors and comb with your left hand.

Hold the scissors with your ring finger in the palm of your hand. Keep your thumb out of the thumb rest until you are ready to cut, and always keep the blades closed. This will prevent you from cutting anything but the hair that you intend on cutting!

Hold the comb in between your thumb and the remaining fingers in the palm of your hand. (See figure 1 below.)

Figure#1

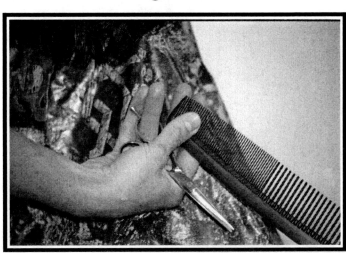

Step#2: You will be combing and sectioning with the hand that you are always holding the scissors in. Now, section the hair with the larger teeth of the comb. By using the larger teeth when sectioning, you will have more control of the hair.

Imagine that the comb is a pencil, and you are drawing a straight line. Create a triangle from the midway point on the top of the head. This will be just above the ears, to no wider than the corner of each eyebrow. (See figure 2 below)

Figure #2

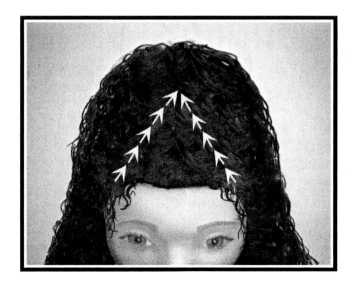

Step#3: After you have created a triangle, comb a small section of hair from the center of the eyebrows, to in between your index and middle finger. This section, also known as your guide, should be no wider than one inch.

When combing any section that you intend on cutting, comb it towards yourself rather than away from yourself.

By combing the hair toward yourself, it will allow you to have more control over the section you are working on. (See figure #3 below.)

Figure#3

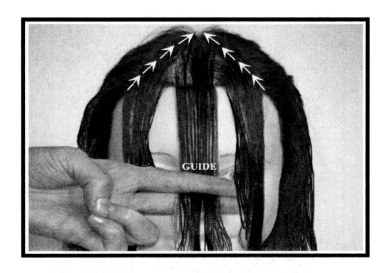

GUIDE

Step#4: Now, slowly transfer the comb from the hand with the scissors, to the opposite hand that is now holding the hair. You will be holding the comb with your index finger and thumb while placing it up and out of your cutting view. You will probably find yourself dropping the comb several times while transferring it from one hand to the other. With a little practice, transferring the comb will become natural. (See figure 4 below.)

Figure #4

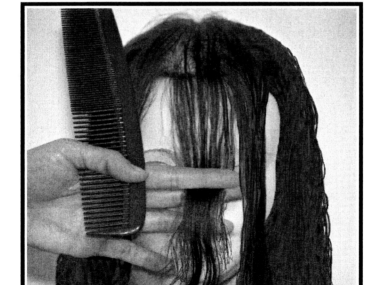

Step#5: Finally, place your thumb in the thumb rest of your scissors. Your thumb will be what primarily controls the scissor blades while you are cutting. (See figure 5 below.)

Figure #5

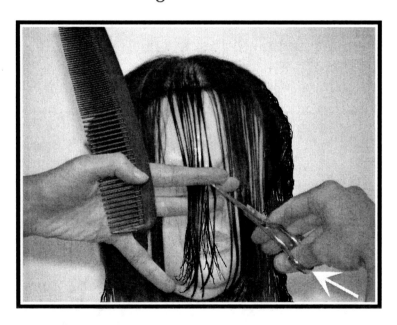

Practice steps 1 through 5 a few times before moving on. Read each step over while studying the photographs. This will prepare you for steps 6 through 8.

After you have practiced the first five steps, you can continue with the remaining steps on the following page.

Remember, only go through the motions of cutting in this chapter, and take your time!

Step#6: Now that your thumb is in the thumb rest of your scissors, and you are holding the hair that you are about to cut; rest the flat side of your scissors in the crease in which you are holding the hair.

While the scissors are resting in the crease of your fingers, slowly open the blades a little at a time. Take your time so that you do not cut yourself. (See figure 6 below.)

Figure #6

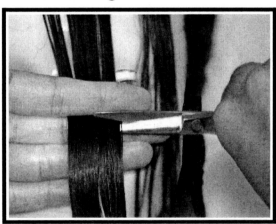

When you are actually cutting in the next chapter, you will be using the crease or line in between your two fingers as a cutting guide. This guide will help you to create a straight line, and it will direct you to and from the direction in which you will be cutting.

Step#7: Go through the motions of cutting the first small section, and then transfer the comb into the same hand that you are holding the scissors.

Starting on one side at the corner of the eyebrow, move towards the center guide. From the center guide, move to the corner of the other eyebrow.

You should be holding the hair in between your index and middle finger, just as you did at the end of step 3.

If you are left handed, you will hold the scissors and comb in the opposite hand. You will also start cutting in the opposite direction. (See figure 7 below.)

Figure#7

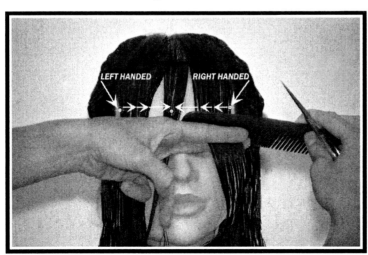

Repeat steps 1 through 7 only going through the motions. After you practice these last few steps over again, you will be ready to move on to chapter 5, "How to Cut the Bangs".

Chapter Five
HOW TO CUT THE BANGS
Two different modifications

Option A: *(the "blunt" look)*

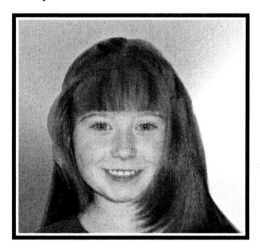

Option B: *(the "tapered" or layered look)*

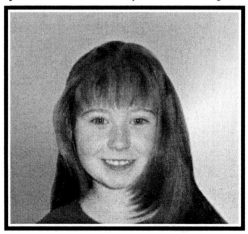

Before starting this chapter, review chapters 2 and 3 very carefully, and then answer the following questions:

✂ *How long do you want the bangs?*

✂ *Do you want the bangs cut blunt? By using this technique, they will look heavier. See option A on page 29.*

✂ *Do you want the bangs cut with "taper" or layers? By using this technique, they will look lighter, and will usually have more volume. See option B on page 29.*

OPTION A: THE BLUNT LOOK

Begin the bang segment by forming a triangle with your comb. Section the hair from just above the ears on the top of the head, to no wider than the corner of each eyebrow. Most everyone's bangs fall naturally in this area. (See figure 1 below.)

Figure #1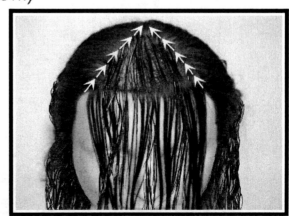

After you form a triangle, study the segment in which you will be cutting. Look for any "cowlicks". These are strong growth patterns where the hair grows out of around different areas of the head. They also make the hair lay in different directions. Everyone has at least one.

Pay special attention to the front hairline. Here especially, it is more noticeable for the hair to shrink after it dries. (See figure 2 below.)

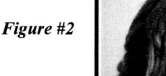

Figure #2

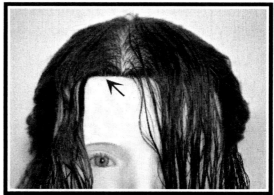

You can cut the bangs dry or wet. If you decide to cut them wet, leave them a little longer than you actually want them after they dry. If you cut them dry, cut them to the exact length that you want. Either way will prevent you from cutting them too short.

To start cutting the bangs, comb a small section from in between the two eyebrows into the center of your index and middle finger. This section should be about one inch wide. While your palm is facing you, focus on the two fingers that are holding the hair.

Releasing the tension on the hair in between your fingers rather than holding it tight, will prevent the hair from shrinking after you cut it.

Comb the hair straight down. Slowly release the tension on it, so that it "springs" up to just where you see it bend: but do not let go. This is about where the bangs are going to be when they dry. (See figure 3 below.)

Figure #3

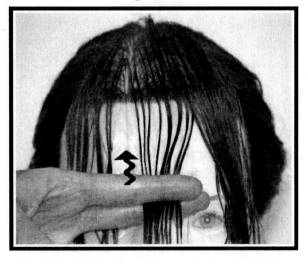

Next, cut this section of hair to the length that you want. This will be your guide, and the halfway point from each eyebrow.

If you hold the scissors with your right hand, start at the corner of the right eyebrow and finish at the corner of the left. If you are left handed, start and finish in the opposite direction. Figure 4 demonstrates the direction that you would start in if you were right handed.

Always align the crease in between your fingers from your starting point to your finishing point. Use your fingers as a straight edge, and keep in mind the length that you have created in the center of the eyebrows. This will guide you through your cut. (See figure 4 below.)

Figure#4

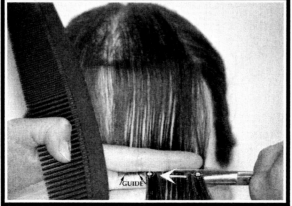

Continue cutting until you reach the corner of the opposite eyebrow. (See figure 5 below.)

Figure #5

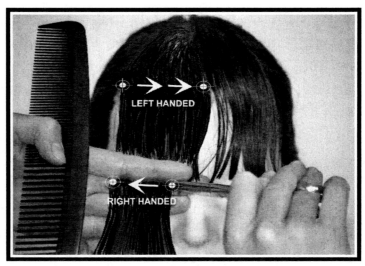

If you cut the bangs while they were wet, dry them before moving on to make sure that they are even. If they are not even, correct them while they are dry.

If you decided that you wanted the blunt look, then leave the bangs just as they are.

If you decided that you wanted the "tapered" or layered look, continue with these last few steps:

OPTION B: (THE "TAPERED" OR LAYERED LOOK)

The word "taper" means that the hair will be slightly layered, which will give the hair in that area a softer look.

After cutting the length of the bangs, horizontally take a section of the triangle and place it in between the crease of your fingers. There will be a small section of hair remaining on the forehead.

If you want the bangs _less dense,_ and _more "tapered" or layered:_

Hold more than half of the hair from this section in between your fingers. Raise this hair a little higher than straight out from the head, and cut. (See figure 6 below.)

 Figure #6

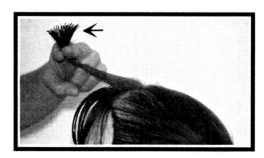

If you choose to make the bangs *more dense,* and *less "tapered"* or *layered:*
Hold less than half of hair from this section in between your fingers, and then proceed to cut. (See figure 7 below.)

Figure #7

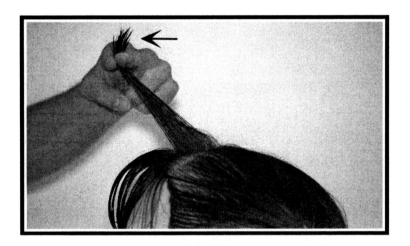

Congratulations! You have now completed the bangs. You can combine this cut with the "All the Same Length Haircut" in the next chapter if you desire.

Chapter Six
HOW TO CUT AN ALL THE SAME LENGTH HAIRCUT
Includes Three Different Modifications

Option A:
(On, or above the shoulders with bangs)

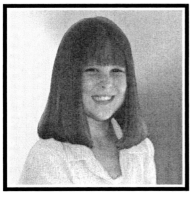

Option B:
(Below the shoulders)

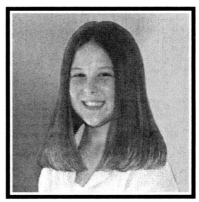

Option C:
(Slightly angled in the front)

Now that you have cut the bangs, you should feel more comfortable holding the scissors and comb together while cutting.

You may need more practice to feel 100% comfortable, so continue to review chapters 2-4 if necessary. The more you practice the steps in chapter 2-4, the more natural haircutting will become.

When you feel ready to begin this chapter, answer the following questions to determine the type of haircut that you want to create:

✄ *Do you want bangs?*

  See option A page 37.

✄ *What length do you want the cut to be? (On, above, or below the shoulders)*

  See option A and B page 37.

✄ *Do you want to add a slight angle in the front to frame the face?*

  See option C page 37.

These questions will help you to determine which steps you are going to take to get your results.

If you answered yes to question 1, "Do you want bangs?" complete the bangs first. Refer back to chapter 5 and treat the bangs as a separate haircut, then move on.

To begin the All The Same Length Haircut, divide the hair into five segments. The hair should be clean and damp.

The term "segments" will be used throughout this book. All five segments will be located in the same area consistently. (See figure 1A and 1B below.)

Figure #1 A
(Left side)

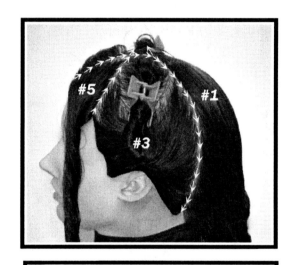

Figure #1 B
(Right side)

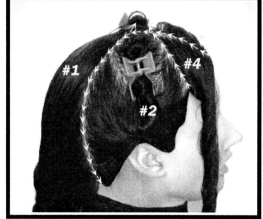

Clip up the following three segments shown on the next few pages. These segments are formed from the top of the head, and will all take the basic shape of triangles.

Start with segment 1. This segment is located at the back of the head. It is formed from the midway point on the top of the head, to where the hairline ends on each side on the back of the neck. (See figure 2 below.)

Figure #2

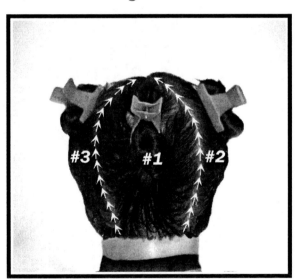

Both segments 2 and 3 begin at the back of the head and continue forward from segment 1. They are formed from the midway point on the top of the head to just above the eyebrows on each side of the head. (See figure 3a and 3b below.)

Figure 3a   *Figure 3b*

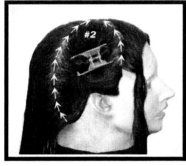 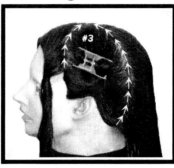

Segments 4 and 5 begin towards the front of the head. They continue forward from segments 2 and 3, and end in the center of the forehead. You will notice that a center part is created in between the two eyebrows. (See figure 4a and 4b below.)

Figure #4a   *Figure #4b*

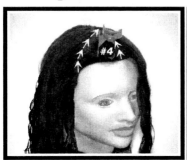 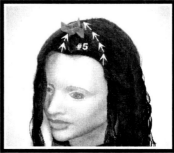

After you divide the hair into the appropriate segments, continue to focus on one segment at a time.

SEGMENT 1:

Start in the back at segment 1. Most everyone's hair has the most density in this area; therefore, you may need to divide this segment into separate horizontal parts to complete the length. This will make it easier for you to cut.

First, divide this segment in half horizontally. Take the top half and clip it up. (See figure 5 below.)

Figure #5

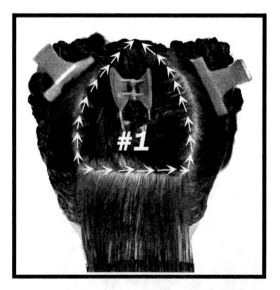

Now, you are going to refer back to your answer to the question in the beginning of this chapter; ("What length do you want the cut to be?")

After you have determined the length, section about 1 inch in width of hair from the very center bottom half of segment 1. As you are holding this hair, make sure that your fingers are resting directly on the skin or back. This will give you a clean cut.

Make sure that the head is facing down towards the floor. This will make it easier for you to see what you are cutting. It will give the back a softer look and slight "undercut." The word undercut means that the hair will go under in a specific area.

Now, cut the center piece to the length that you want. (See figure 6 below.)

Figure #6

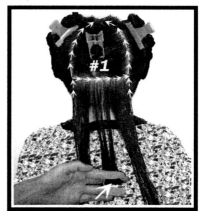

Remember:

>< *The hand with the most dexterity should be holding the scissors.*

>< *The back of your fingers should be resting on the skin or back while holding the hair.*

>< *The head should be facing down towards the floor.*

>< *Your fingers and the crease in between them, will guide you to and from the direction in which you are cutting. Imagine that you are "connecting the dots."*

>< *Focus on the crease in between your fingers making sure it is straight, and aligned with the "dots" that you are connecting to and from.*

Take the piece of hair that you just cut, and use this as your guide.

To complete the first horizontal section, cut from one side to the other. The side that you start from will depend on which hand that you are holding the scissors in. Your scissors will always be pointing to the center guide. (See figure 7 below.)

Figure#7

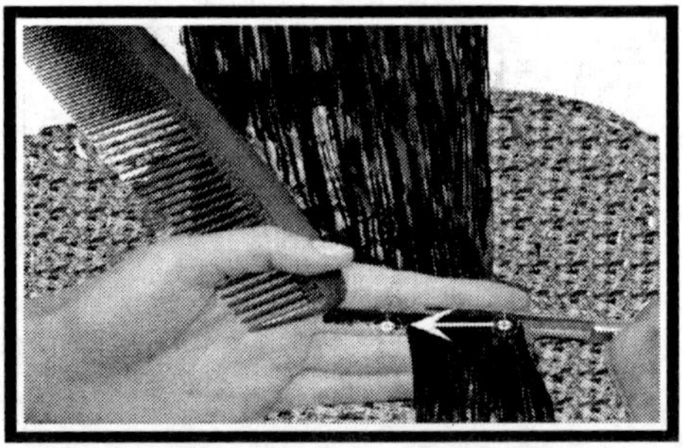

Now, check this section to make sure that it is even. Take your comb and place it below the length. Hold the comb horizontally and look for balance. (See figure 8a below.)

Figure #8a

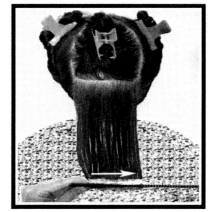

Complete segment one, by bringing the remainder of hair down, and cutting it all to the same length. (See figure 8b below.) If you can't see your guide, continue to bring down as many horizontal sections needed to do so.

Figure #8b

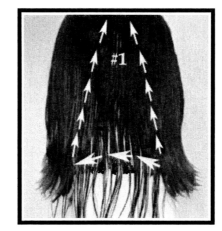

CHECKING SEGMENT ONE

Check segment one by re-combing all the segments straight down from where they were cut. First, use the wide then narrow teeth of the comb. This will allow you to remove any unwanted hairs before and after the hair dries. These hairs are caused by inconsistent growth patterns, or from the head not being in the same position throughout the cut. Check again for balance.

SEGMENTS 2 AND 3:

You are now ready to move on to the sides of the head. These options will allow you to create three different looks in the front. Before moving on, you will need to refer back to your answers to the remaining questions in the beginning of this chapter.

OPTION A: "Is the length resting on, above or below the shoulders?" (See options A, B, and C on page 37.)

OPTION B: "Do you want the front to be the same length as the back?" (See option A and B on page 37.)

OPTION C: "Do you want a slight angle in the front?" (See option C on page 37.)

OPTION A: BACK LENGTH RESTING ON OR ABOVE THE SHOULDERS AND FRONT LENGTH SAME AS BACK

Remember:

✂ *Your fingers and the crease in between them will guide you to and from the direction in which you are cutting. Imagine that you are "connecting the dots."*

✂ *Focus on the crease in between your fingers making sure that it is straight and aligned with the "dots" that you are connecting to and from.*

SEGMENT 2:

After you complete segment one, begin at segment 2. If the hair is resting on or above the shoulders and you want the length the same as the back:

Connect segments 2 and 1 together by resting the ear on the opposite shoulder that you are cutting.

Rest the back of your fingers on the neck. This will make it easier for you to see what you are cutting, and it will allow you to create a clean straight line. (See figure 9 below.)

Figure #9

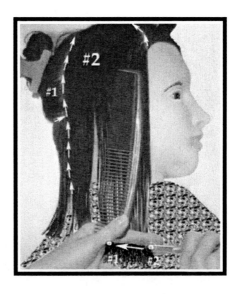

After you complete segment 2, go to segment 3. Complete this segment in the same manner as you did segment 2, by connecting it with segment 1. (See figure 10 below.)

Figure #10

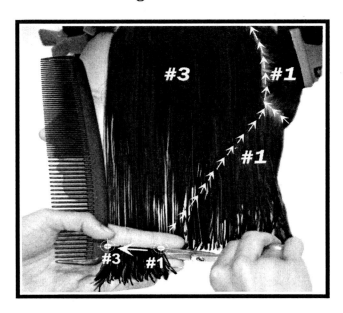

SEGMENTS 4 AND 5:

To complete the front of this haircut, unfasten segments 4 and 5. In this case, the length of these last two segments will be the same length as segment 2 and 3.

Start segment 4 by connecting it with segment 2. Keep the head in the same position so that the ear is resting on the shoulder of the opposite side that you are cutting. Note that the fingers are lined up with the length of segment 2. (See figure 11 below).

Figure #11

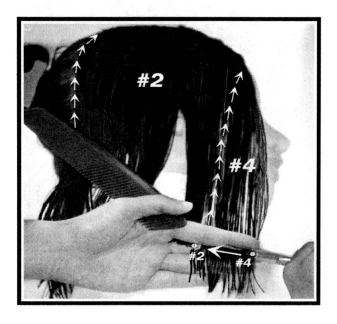

After connecting segments 4 and 2, connect 3 and 5 in the same manner. (See figure 12 below.)

Figure #12

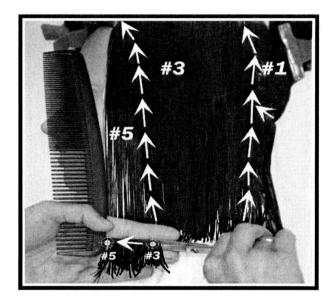

CHECKING THE FRONT:

Now, stand in front and position the head so that it is straight and facing forward. Use any level surface as your guide to make sure that both sides are even. (See figure 13 below.)

Figure #13

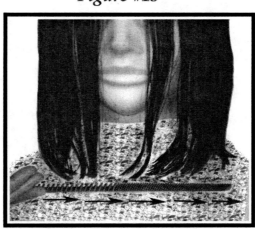

RECHECK THE ENTIRE CUT:

After you check the front, recheck the entire haircut. Dry the cut until it is slightly damp. This will allow you to see what the cut will look like after it is almost dry. Remember, hair shrinks up after it is dry, so you want to make sure the cut is still even from this perspective.

Recheck the back (refer to page 46). Now, recheck the sides *and* front using the same technique on page 36 and above.

OPTION B: BACK LENGTH RESTING BELOW SHOULDERS AND FRONT LENGTH SAME AS BACK

If the length is below the shoulders, and you want the front to be the same length as the back:

Complete segment one, by cutting it to the appropriate length. Then, complete the sides by connecting segments 2 and 1 together.

Turn the head so that the chin is just above the shoulder of the side that you are cutting.

Use the surface of the back to cut on. This will make it easier for you to see your guides, and to cut a clean straight line. (See figure 14 below.)

Figure #14

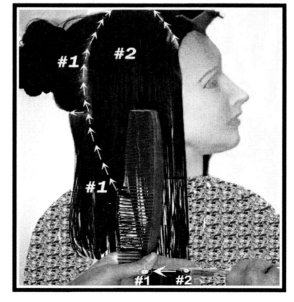

After you complete segment 2, go to segment 3. Complete this segment in the same manner as you did segment 2, connecting it with segment 1. (See figure 15 below.)

Figure #15

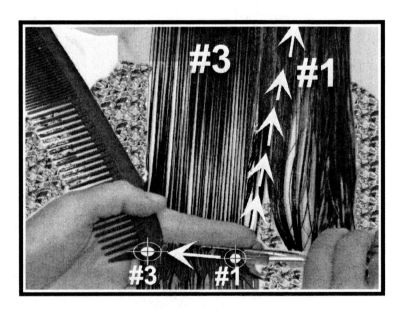

SEGMENTS 4 AND 5:

To complete the front of this haircut, connect segments 4 and 2 together. Keep the head in the same position with the chin just above the shoulder. (See figure 16 below.)

Figure #16

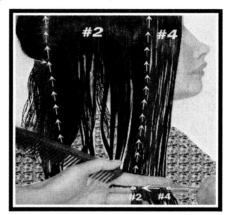

Now, connect segments 3 and 5 together. (See figure 17 below).

Figure #17

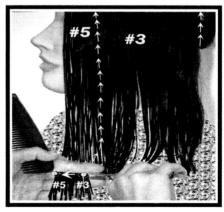

To check this haircut refer back to page 52.

OPTION C: FRONT SLIGHTLY ANGLED TO FRAME THE FACE WITH ADDED VOLUME AND TAPER *(Front will be no shorter than just below the chin)*

Remember:

✂ *Your fingers and the crease in between them, will guide you to and from the direction in which you are cutting. Imagine that you are "connecting the dots".*

✂ *Focus on the crease in between your fingers making sure that it is straight and aligned with the "dots" that you are connecting to and from.*

This technique will not create a drastic change in the front length. It will add a small amount of fullness and more style to the entire cut. I recommend that this haircut should only be used on hair that is in good condition on the ends of the bottom length. This will allow you to see the correct guides accurately. For example, it is very common among young children who are getting first time haircuts, to have fine, straggly, and uneven hair at the bottom length. This type of hair will make it harder for you to see your guide. If this is the case, I would suggest cutting this hair to a healthy length when you are cutting the back. It is possible that you may have to remove between 1 to 2 inches. Although, after you remove this, it will give the hair more fullness and will allow it to grow out more evenly. This hair will also become denser as the child grows older.

To obtain a maximum amount of volume with this cut, I recommend that the length in the Back be just above the shoulders or no longer than the shoulder blades.

If you chose option C, and want the front slightly angled and "tapered", complete segments 1 through 3 first. Follow the correct procedures in the beginning of this chapter according to the chosen length.

By using this technique on the front, you will create a small amount of taper at the same time.

Remember, the word "taper" means that the hair in that area will have a slight layer to it. Being that the hair will be slightly layered or cut at different lengths, it will also have more volume.

After completing segments 1 through 3, begin the front.

Section the hair from the top of the head to just in front of the ears on both sides. (See figure 18 below.)

Figure #18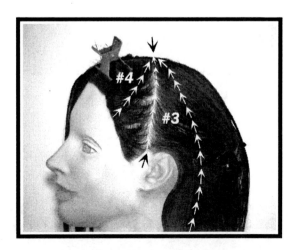

Unfasten the hair that you just sectioned in front of the ears (segments 4, 5 and half of 2 and 3). Clip the remaining hair up and out of your way.

Next, cut a guide no shorter than just below the chin and no wider than one inch in between segments 4 and 5. (See figure 19 below.)

Figure #19

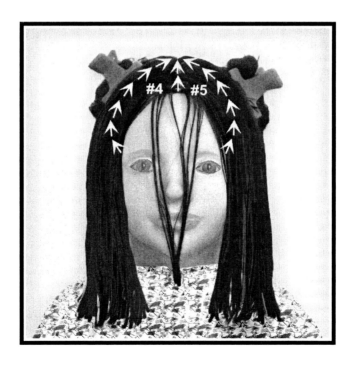

Connect the guide that you just cut, with the length of the hair that you sectioned in front of the ear.

Rest the ear on the opposite shoulder that you are cutting, and pull all of this hair forward towards you. Be fully aware of where your two guides are. (See figure #20 below.)

Figure #20

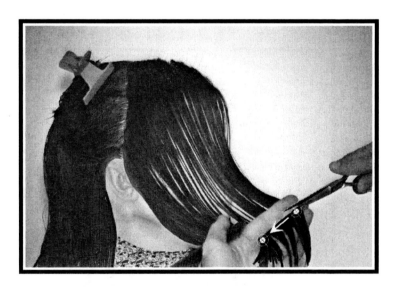

After you complete one side, complete the other in the same manner. (See figure 21 below).

Figure #21

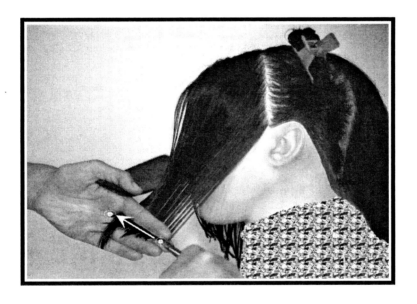

Check the cut to make sure that it is balanced. Refer back to page 52 if necessary.

You have now completed The All The Same Length Haircut! By now, you are probably comfortable enough to move on to the next cut. If not, simply review chapters 2-4 again.

Before beginning the next chapter, you must clearly understand chapters 2 and 3, which focus on "cowlicks" and the front hairline.

Chapter Seven
HOW TO CUT SHORT LAYERS INTO THE HAIR

An above the Ears and Collar Haircut that can be Modified to Different Lengths

Option A:
(Above the ears and collar with less bulk)

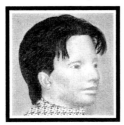

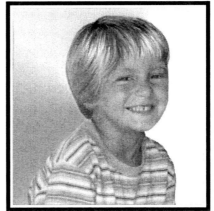

Option B:
(Covering _the_ ears with more _bulk)_

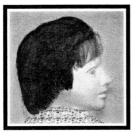

By cutting layers into the hair, you can create many different looks.

The more layers that you cut into the hair, the shorter the hair will become in that area. The bulk or weight in that area will also be reduced. (See option A on page 63.)

The fewer layers that you cut into the hair, the longer the hair in that area will remain. It will also contain more bulk or weight. (See option B on page 63.)

Before you begin this cut answer the following questions:

✂ *Do you want the sides above the ears or covering them?*

✂ *Do you want the cut to have more bulk or less bulk?*

This book will primarily focus on a cut that is above the ears and collar with less bulk. (See option A on page 63.)

You can achieve the longer look (option B), with a few simple modifications. I will explain how to modify it later on in this chapter.

OPTION A: ABOVE THE EARS AND COLLAR WITH LESS BULK

You will be dividing the hair into 6 segments. The first 5 segments are located in the same area that they were in chapter six. Refer back to chapter six on page 39 if needed.

Remember all 5 segments are in the basic shapes of triangles, and they each begin from the midway point at the top of the head.

Before you start, make sure that the hair is clean and damp.

Begin with segment 1. After you divide it into its proper location, cut the length. Start at the bottom of this segment in the very center. Cut a piece of hair about 1 inch wide above the collar or just below the hairline. Be careful not to cut above the hairline. Most people do not like it cut that short unless it is specified. (See figure 1 below.)

Figure #1

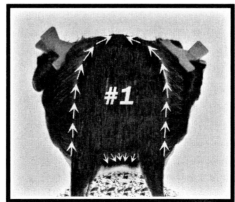

Remember:

✂ *The side that you start cutting from will depend on which hand that you hold the scissors in to cut.*

✂ *The back of your fingers should be resting on the skin while holding the hair. It is not recommended to cut the hair directly on the skin until you feel 100% comfortable with this cut. Doing this could cause you to cut the skin if you are not careful.*

✂ *The head should be facing down toward the floor.*

✂ *Your fingers and the crease in between them will guide you to and from the direction in which you are cutting. Imagine that you are "connecting the dots."*

✂ *Focus on the crease in between your two fingers making sure that it is straight, and aligned with the "dots" that you are connecting to and from.*

Complete segment 1, by cutting from one side to the other. (See figure 2 below).

Figure #2

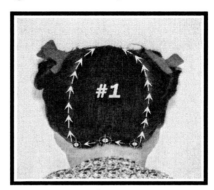

Now, divide the hair into segments 2 and 3. Refer back top chapter 6 page 41 if needed.

Begin segment 2 by holding a piece of hair about 1 inch wide where the hairline stops in front of the ear. Cut this to right above the ears. Be careful not to cut above the hairline. Rest the ear on the opposite shoulder of the side that you are cutting. This will make it easier for you to see what you are doing. (See figure 3 below.)

Figure #3

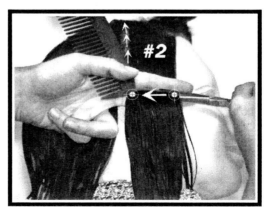

Complete segment 2 by connecting its length to segment 1. Again, be careful not to cut above the hairline. You may need to push the ear out of the way to remove any hairs that are out of place. Continue to rest the ear on the opposite side in which you are cutting. (See figure 4 below.)

Figure #4

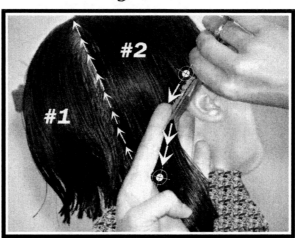

Remember:

✂ *The segment that you start at will depend on the hand that you are holding the scissors in.*

✂ *Imagine that you are "connecting the dots".*

✂ *Focus on the crease in between your fingers, making sure that it is straight and aligned with the "dots" that you are connecting to and from.*

After completing segment 2, go to segment 3. Complete this segment in the same manner as you did segment 2.

Cut a 1 inch wide piece of hair where the hairline stops in front of the ear. Then connect segments 3 and 1 together. (See figure 5 below.)

Figure #5

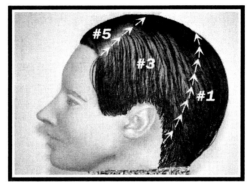

Now, you can continue to divide segments 4 and 5 (refer to page 41 if needed).

These two segments should be tackled very carefully. They are located where the receding area is on the forehead and the front hairline. This is where the hair has the least amount of density. It also may contain many different "cowlicks"; therefore, you will need to be fully aware of not cutting this area too short. To prevent this from happening, leave the hair in these two segments longer than you actually want it.

To begin segment's 4 and 5, take a piece of hair about 1 inch wide in the center of both segments (which is also the center of the forehead and bang area).

Before you cut this to the length that you want the bangs, comb the hair straight down. Slowly release the tension on it so that it "springs" up to just where you see it bend, but do not let go. This is just about where the bangs are going to be when they dry. (See figure 6 below.)

Figure #6

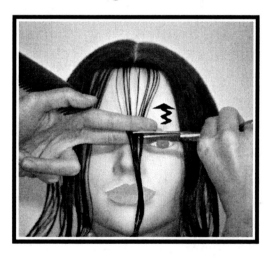

After you have determined how short that you want the bangs, cut the 1 inch wide piece of hair to that length.

Complete segment 4, by connecting from the length that you've just created in the center, with segment 2.

Connect these two segments very carefully by directing the hair forward towards yourself. Depending on how long the hair was in this area, there may not be too much hair to remove.

You may need to create an imaginary line as you are directing it forward. This will prevent you from cutting the hair too short in between these two points. Only focus on the hair that is in between this imaginary line. Release the tension until the hair "springs" up, but do not let go. Now, proceed to cut. (See figure 7 below).

Figure #7

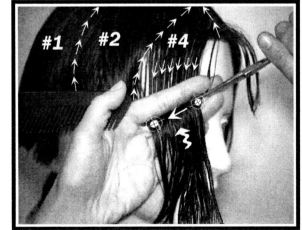

Next, go to segment 5 and use the same technique to connect it with segment 3. (See figure 8 below.)

Figure #8

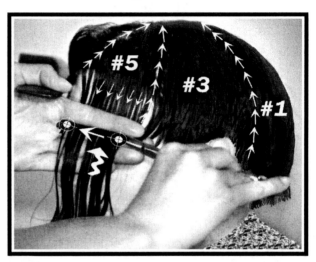

Remember:

✂ _Leave the hair extra long in this area._

✂ _Comb the hair forward towards you into an imaginary line._

✂ _Release the tension until the hair "springs" up, but do not let go; then, proceed to cut._

These tips will prevent you from cutting the hair too short in this area.

After you finish segments 4 and 5, you will have completed the entire length around the head.

The next step is to divide the hair into segment 6. This segment is located at the entire top section of the head. This is what will provide the guide for the length of the layers.

The width of this segment will be about 3 to 4 inches, depending on the shape at the top of the head.

The length will start from the very back top of the head to the front hairline. (See figure 9 below.)

Figure#9

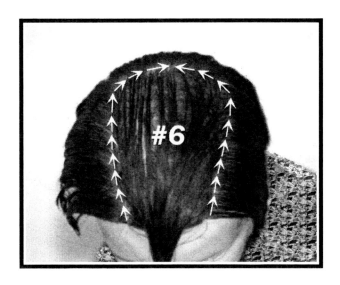

After you divide the hair into segment 6, you must locate any "cowlicks" which may be present. Study the hair just below this segment all the way around the head.

You will probably find more than one "cowlick", but your main objective should be to find the biggest or strongest one. This is usually located in the back of the head at the top part of segment 1.

To locate this "cowlick", look for where the hair is growing in different directions. This area may also look very thin and the scalp may be showing. The hair in this area may already be sticking up, or close to it. Locating this will help you to determine a guide to prevent you from cutting the hair too short.

Finding "cowlicks" will become more natural with experience. (See figure 10 below.)

Figure #10

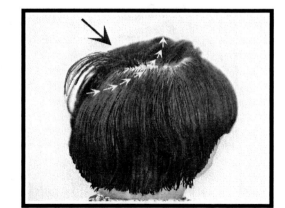

Once you locate the "cowlick" in segment 1, use it as a guide to start creating the length in segment 6.

Take a piece of hair from the "cowlick"(about 1 inch wide), and lift it straight up towards the ceiling.

With the scissors resting on top of your fingers, cut this guide as short as it will go without sticking up. Cut it a little at a time, so that it still lies on the head. If it is already sticking up, do not cut it any shorter. (See figure 11 below.)

Figure#11

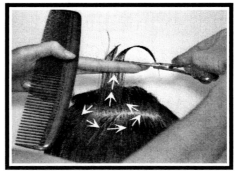

After you cut this, keep it visible. Twist it together so that you can use it as a guide to cut the rest of the segment. (See figure 12 below.)

Figure#12

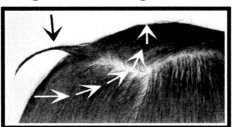

Continue with segment 6. Create a vertical section no wider than 1 inch from the very center of this segment. Begin cutting it from the length of the bangs, to the guide that you just cut in the back of the head. Connect these two "dots" together. (See figure 13 below.)

Figure #13

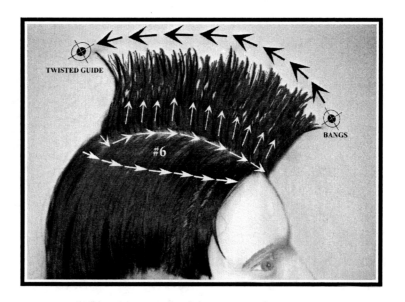

After you cut the vertical center section, you will use this as your guide to complete segment 6.

Begin at the top back part of the head.

Create a horizontal part from each side of segment 6, and some of the vertical center section that you just cut.

Extend, or over-direct the hair that you are holding forward towards the front. This will maintain the length in this area so that it doesn't stick up.

With the scissors resting on top of your fingers, remove the longer hair here to match the length of the hair in the vertical center section. (See figure 14 below.)

Figure #14

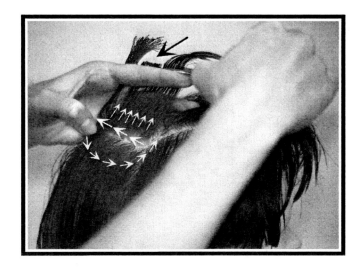

Continue forward to the front.

To do this, take another horizontal part, including the last part that you just cut and the vertical center section. Hold this straight up to the ceiling, rather than over directing it forward. Now, cut it to the same length. Remember to cut on top of your fingers. Make sure that your fingers are horizontally straight. (See figure 15 below.)

Figure #15

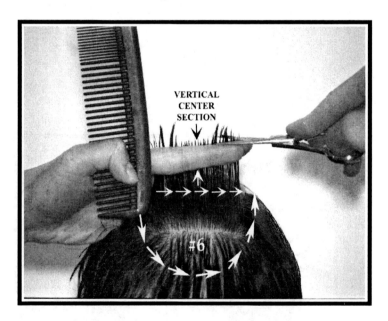

Continue this same procedure until you reach the very front where the receding area starts. This should be right where segments 4 and 5 begin.

Instead of holding these last few segments straight up to the ceiling to cut, extend them or "over direct" them all towards the back of the head. Let some of the bang length fall out onto the forehead. This will maintain the length in these last few sections, and prevent you from cutting the hair too short. There should not be much hair to remove here. (See figure 16 below).

Figure #16

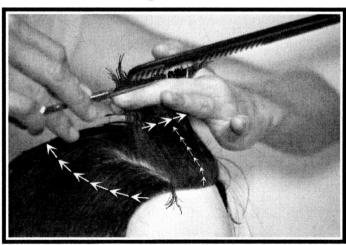

Segment 6 is now complete. You will use this as your top guide to cut the layers.

To begin the layers, divide the hair into the first 5 segments. Refer back to page 39 if needed.

Rewet the hair and put conditioner in it to make the hair easier to work with.

Complete one segment at a time. Each one will be divided by its own guide in the center. This will make it easier for you and will keep you organized. It will also allow you cut certain segments shorter than others while still keeping the haircut balanced. For example, some people like their sides shorter with less weight and their back longer with more weight. In this case, you would remove more hair from the sides than the back. With this technique, you will have no problem blending these segments together.

CUTTING THE LAYERS IN SEGMENT 1:
Remember:

✂ *Cut on top of your fingers.*

✂ *Your fingers and the crease in between them will guide you to and from the direction that you are cutting. Imagine that you are "connecting the dots". There are two "dots" to be aware of; the bottom length and the top length of segment 6.*

✂ _Focus on the crease in between your fingers. Make sure that it is straight and aligned with what you are connecting to and from._

Begin at segment 1. Cut a vertical guide in the center of this segment. Use the length of segment 6 and the length that you created on the bottom for your two guides. Start at the bottom length and connect up to segment 6.
When cutting, comb the hair straight out from the head. Begin by letting some of the bottom length fall out of your fingers. This will prevent you from cutting a hole into the bottom. (See figure 17 below.)

Figure #17

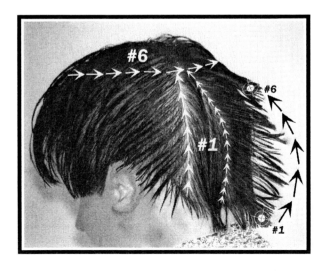

After you create the guide for segment 1, continue to cut vertical sections from this guide to each corner of this segment.

Position yourself so that you can comfortably connect from the bottom length up to segment 6.

Moving to one side, pick up another vertical section including part of the center guide that you just cut. By including part of this guide, it will allow you to consistently remove all of the hair.

Before you cut, let some of the bottom length fall out.

Complete the first half of segment 1. (See figure 18 below.)

Figure #18

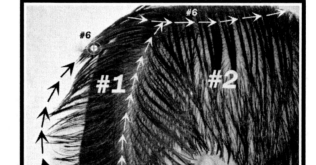

To complete the second half of segment 1, start at the center guide again. Pick up a part of this guide and move toward the opposite corner. Comb the hair straight out from the head, letting some of the bottom length fall out of your fingers.

Cut on top of your fingers and connect from the bottom length up to segment 6. (See figure 19 below.

Figure #19

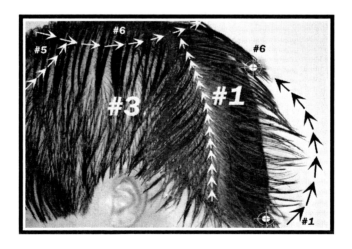

You have now completed segment 1. (See figure 20 below.)

Figure #20

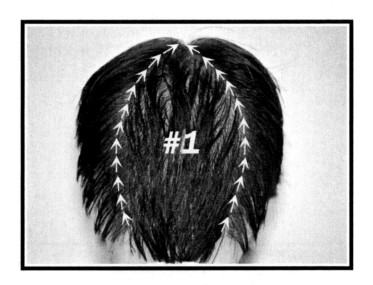

CUTTING THE LAYERS IN SEGMENTS 2 AND 3:

Remember:

✂ *Your fingers and the crease in between them will guide you to and from the direction that you are cutting. Imagine that you are "connecting the dots".*

✂ *Focus on the crease in between your fingers. Make sure that it is straight and aligned with what you are connecting to and from.*

To begin segments 2 and 3, you will still use the top guide from segment 6, and the bottom length.

SEGMENT 2:

Beginning at segment 2 and create a guide in the center by taking a vertical section just on top of the ear. Connect from the bottom length up to segment 6 just as you did when you cut the layers in segment 1 on page 80 and 81. (See figure 21 below.)

Figure #21

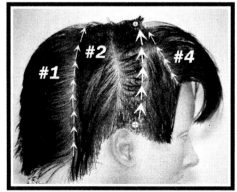

Move from the center guide to the corner of segment 1. Remember to always include part of the previous section that you just cut. This will allow you to consistently remove all the hair.

Cut on top of your fingers connecting from the bottom to the top.

When you get to segment 1, you will need to blend it with segment 2. To do this, take part of segment 1 and part of segment 2 together and create a vertical section. Comb this section straight out from the head, and connect from the bottom length up to segment 6. This will blend segments 1 and 2 together. (See figure 22 below.)

Figure #22

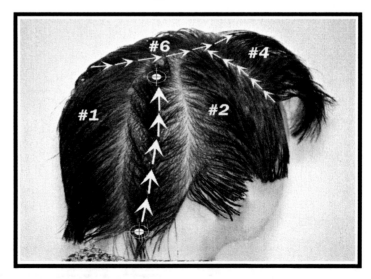

To complete the other half of segment 2, pick up part of the center guide and continue cutting to in front of the ear right before the corner of the eyebrow.

Comb this hair straight out from the head. With the scissors resting on top of your fingers, connect from the bottom length up to segment 6.

Do not go beyond the corner of the eyebrow at this time. This will prevent you from cutting into segment 4, which is where the receding area starts on this side. (See figure 23 below.)

Figure #23

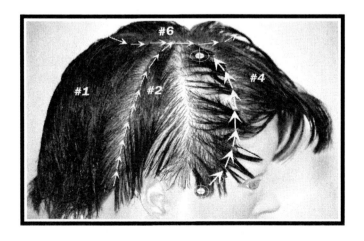

SEGMENT 3:

Complete segment 3 using the same procedure as you used to complete segment 2.

Create a vertical center guide just as you did in figure 21 on page 85. Move from the center guide to the corner of segment 1. Blend segment 3 with segment 1 by combining both segments and combing the hair straight out from the head.

Now, connect from the bottom length up to segment 6. (See figure 24 below.)

Figure #24

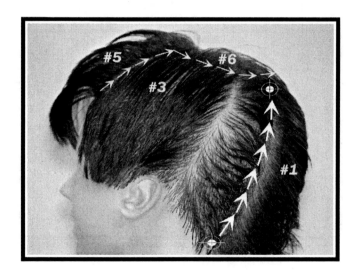

To complete the other half of segment 3, begin at the center guide. Combine this with your next vertical section as you move to in front of the ear just before the corner of the eyebrow.

DO NOT go beyond the corner of the eyebrow. This will prevent you from cutting into segment 5 which is where the receding area starts on this side. (See figure 25 below.)

Figure #25

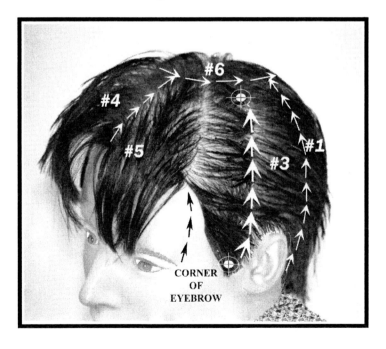

CUTTING THE LAYERS IN SEGMENTS 4 AND 5:

Remember:

✂ *Your fingers and the crease in between them will guide you to and from the direction in which you are cutting. Imagine that you are "connecting the dots".*

✂ *Focus on the crease in between your fingers. Make sure that it is straight and aligned with what you are connecting to and from.*

Again, segments 4 and 5 need to be handled with care because they are located where the receding area is. There also may be cowlicks here. There should not be much hair coming off of these last two segments.

For these last 2 segments, you will use segment 6 as your guide only. Let the bottom length fall out of your fingers so that you don't cut a hole into this area.

SEGMENT 4:

Begin at segment 4. This is located in front of segment 2, which is where the hairline stops in front of the ear.

Using segment 6 as your only guide, take a vertical section where segment 4 begins.

Rather than combing this hair straight out from the head, comb it straight up to the ceiling. Your fingers should be horizontal and still holding your guide at segment 6. The bottom length should fall out of your fingers. Cut the remaining hair in between your fingers straight across.

You may only need to take one horizontal section in segment 4. It will depend on the amount of hair in this area. Continue to the end of segment 4 which is located at the center of the forehead. Remember, there shouldn't be much hair to remove here. (See figure 26 below.)

Figure #26

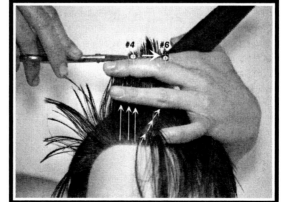

SEGMENT 5:

Now, complete segment 5. This is located in the same area as segment 4, but on the opposite side of the head. Follow the same procedure as you did in segment 4 on page 91.

Remember that you will be using segment 6 as your guide only. The bottom length will fall out of your fingers.

Make sure that your fingers are horizontal and that you are holding part of segment 6 before you cut.

Use the same amount of vertical sections that you did in segment 4.

When you get ready to cut, there should not be much hair to remove in this segment. (See figure 27 below).

Figure #27

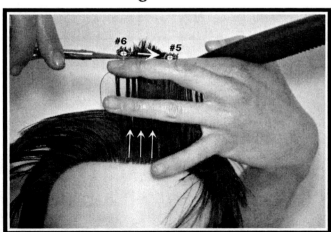

HOW TO MODIFY THE LENGTH AND LAYERS IF NECESSARY:

You can modify this same haircut to any length that you want. Follow these simple steps if you want the hair *SHORTER:*

Do not cut segment 6 any shorter unless you want the hair here to stick up.

First, cut the **length** shorter, by following the steps on pages 65-72. Do not go any shorter than above the ears in segments 2 and 3.

Then, cut the **layers** shorter, by following the steps on pages 80-92. This time remove more hair in between the bottom length and segment 6. To remove more hair from the bottom length and segment 6, hold your fingers closer to the head. Position the head forward closer to the floor to make it easier for you to grab more hair.

Continue on with the same cutting procedures to complete the haircut, but remember to keep the angle of your fingers consistent. (See figure 28 below.)

Figure #28

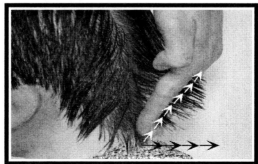

Follow these simple steps if you want the cut to be *LONGER:*

Leave the **length** longer if desired by following the steps on pages 65-72.

To maintain the length of the **layers**, remove less hair by following the same procedure for cutting the layers on pages 80-92. Let more of the bottom length fall out of your fingers.

Continue on with the same cutting procedures to complete the haircut. Remember to keep the angle of your fingers consistent and let the same amount of hair fall out of your fingers around the entire bottom of the head (preferably 1 - 2 inches). (See figure 29 below.)

Figure #29

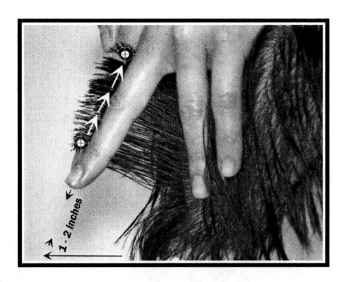

HOW TO CHECK THE SHORT LAYERED CUT:

There are many different ways to check this haircut. I recommend using more than one way in the beginning. Once you feel confident enough to know that your cuts are balanced, you can get by with checking your cut by using one procedure only.

First, stand in front to check for overall balance. Then, take a large arced section from one side to the other. Stand behind the head and comb the hair straight out from it. This will allow you to see if the hair on both sides of the head is even. (See figure 30 below.)

Figure #30

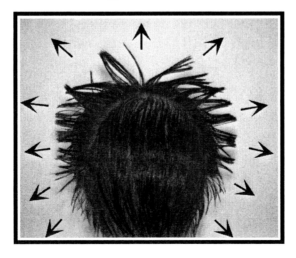

You can also check through the haircut by going through it in the same or opposite direction that you cut it. For example, only go through the motions of cutting by repeating the steps on pages 81-92. Or, go through the same cutting motions but start at segment 5 and end at segment 4. You could also start at segment 4 and end at segment 5. Either way will allow you to see any longer hairs that you may have missed.

Be consistent when checking. Make sure that you are holding the hair in your fingers the same way that you cut it. You should be able to see your original cutting pattern. The cutting line should look clean, with no longer straggly hairs beyond it.

If you do find longer hairs or the hair in a specific area is not balanced, adjust that area to the correct length. If you have to adjust the entire segment, simply repeat the procedure for that segment.

When checking, DO NOT RE-CUT YOUR ORIGINAL HAIRCUT! "If it isn't broken, don't fix it."

I recommend using two of the procedures on this page until you are 100% comfortable.

After you check the haircut and make any necessary adjustments, use your clippers to cut the sideburns to the desired length. If you own a pair of trimmers, use them.

When you use clippers for trimming the sideburns, use the blade that is already attached; or attach the blade that cuts the shortest. (See figure 31 below.)

Figure #31

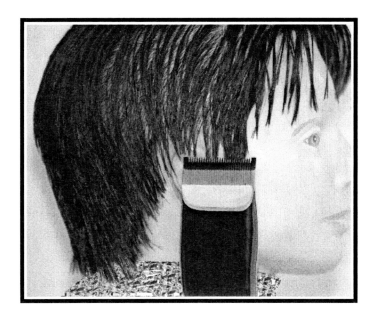

Now, clean up any unwanted hairs behind the ears and on the back of the neck to complete this haircut. (See figure 32 below.)

Figure #32

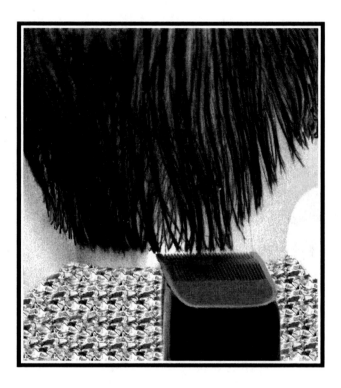

Congratulations! You now know how to cut layers into the hair. This is a very common haircut among both male and female in any age group.

You can now move on to chapter eight, and learn to confidently use a pair of clippers!

Chapter Eight
USING CLIPPERS
All the Information Needed to Begin this Cut, and to Modify it to any Length that You Desire

Option A
(All the same length)

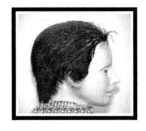

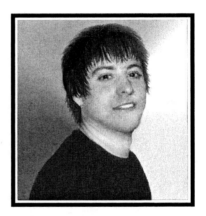

Option B:
(Longer top with shorter sides and back) "faded"

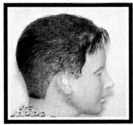

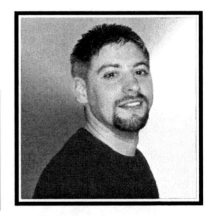

Clippers are tools that are used to remove large amounts of hair; usually more than you can remove with your scissors. With some haircuts, clippers are used for efficiency.

Many people are uncomfortable when they first use clippers because they are unaware of how much hair that is going to come off. You will be surprised at how easy it actually is!

After reading this chapter, you will feel very comfortable using clippers. You will also be happy to know that there is no need to visit a barber shop or salon for this simple and quick haircut!

Before using clippers, you will need to have some idea of how they function. There are many makes and models of clippers as I briefly explained in chapter one.

Most of the least expensive models have non detachable metal blades with plastic guards that attach to them. The plastic guards are used to create different lengths of hair.

Usually, the most expensive models come with a detachable metal blade that the plastic guards attach to. If this blade is used directly on the skin with no plastic guard, it will remove all of the hair on the head.

You can purchase a variety of different sized metal blades to use directly on the skin. Even though they are more expensive than the plastic guards, they do give you a much cleaner cut.

Unless you are already very experienced with clippers, I recommend using the plastic guards to begin with. They are a lot less expensive and they make blending much easier if you are a beginner.

Whichever brand you choose to purchase, the plastic guards are pretty close to the same size.

You will find the information that you need relating to plastic guards on the following page.

All or some of the following sizes are included in most of the clipper sets that you can purchase. These guards can also be purchased separately. It is important to purchase every size available. This will give you more variety.

> *1/8 of an inch*
> *¼ of an inch*
> *3/8 of an inch*
> *½ of an inch*
> *¾ of an inch*
> *5/8 of an inch*
> *7/8 of an inch*
> *1 inch*
> *1 ¼ inches*

Most of the sizes are labeled directly on the plastic guard or on the package insert. It is good to familiarize yourself with the sizes of these guards. Some stylists and clients refer to the guards as numbers going from the smallest to the largest.

For example: The 1/8 of an inch guard could be recognized as a #1; while a 1¼ inch guard could be recognized as a #9.

If you want to obtain of visual of what the length of the hair is going to actually look like before cutting it, take a small ruler and measure the length of the plastic guard straight out from the base of the scalp. (See figure 1 below.)

Figure #1

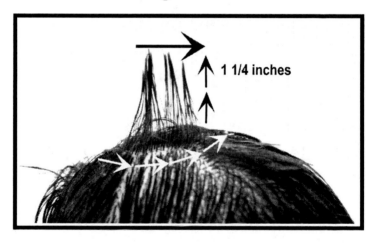

This is an example of the guard which is 1¼ inches long.

Here are certain points to be aware of before you begin a clipper cut:

✂ *Make sure the hair is clean and free from heavy gels or hairsprays. The hair will not cut consistently when dirty.*

✂ *When using certain brands of clippers, the hair must be dry. You could risk electrical shock if the hair is wet. Always read the manual included with your clippers.*

✂ *Clippers will remove the hair more efficiently when the hair is dry. When the hair is wet, the blades push the hair rather than cut it.*

✂ *Drying the hair will allow you to see "cowlicks" and other growth patterns a lot easier. When you do encounter cowlicks, clipper these areas in the opposite direction in which they grow. This will be the only way to remove this hair.*

✂ *If you are using clippers for the first time, the safest thing to do is to start out with the longest guard. If you do this, you will not have to worry about going too short. It will allow you to go shorter a little at a time and also get the feel for the different lengths.*

✂ *Always hold the plastic guard securely as you clipper the hair to prevent the guard from falling off.*

Now that you have read the important points on clipper cutting, you can begin the cut!

Before you begin removing the hair with clippers, you will need to have an idea of how short that you want it. Remember, if you are not sure begin with the longest guard first.

Decide on what length you want the haircut to be and then move on with the following procedures:

A: ALL THE SAME LENGTH

To create a clipper cut that is all the same length, simply start out by clipping the entire head with the longest guard. If this guard is not short enough, continue on with the next shortest guard.

Complete the cut by following the procedures on pages 117 and 118.

B: LONGER TOP WITH SHORTER SIDES AND BACK "faded"

This cut can be modified to any length just by changing the size of the guards.

First, select the longest guard that you have. Remember, if you want to obtain a visual of the length before cutting it, measure the length of the guard that you selected straight out from the base of the scalp. (See page 101.)

Attach the guard to your clippers the proper way. Make sure that it is secured tightly onto the correct metal blade.

This book is going to demonstrate a cut starting with the guard that is 1¼ inches long.

Begin this cut by turning the switch on, and resting the *entire* surface of the plastic guard on the head. The plastic guard will not cut the hair any shorter than its identified length. So, don't hesitate when you have a plastic guard attached, because it will protect you from removing too much hair.

Clipper the entire head with the guard labeled 1¼ inch. Be aware of cowlicks and remember to clip them in the opposite direction in which they grow. You may need to clip around this area a couple times in all directions. This will ensure that you have removed all the hair. (See figure 2 below.)

Figure #2

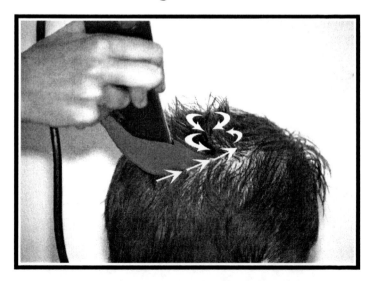

After you have clipped the entire head of hair with the 1¼ inch guard, remove it and attach the ¾ of an inch guard. This guard is still long enough to blend easily with the first guard that you used. At this time, you don't have to necessarily follow the order of using the 1 inch, 7/8 of an inch, then 5/8 of an inch before using the ¾ of an inch guard.

Stand on one side and place the thumb of the hand that is not holding the clippers, just above the eyebrows. This will be the highest point to where you will clip the hair for now.

Use your thumb as your guide. Start on one side and clip up to your thumb. When you reach your thumb, clip the hair away from the head and towards yourself. Take your time to remove all of this hair. If you continue this technique slowly, it will allow you to easily blend the longer hair on top to the shorter hair that you are clipping. (See figure 3 below.)

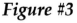 *Figure #3*

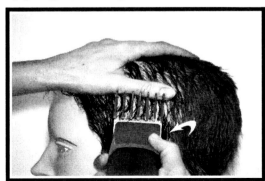

Now repeat the same procedure on the opposite side of the head. (See figure #4 below.)

Figure #4

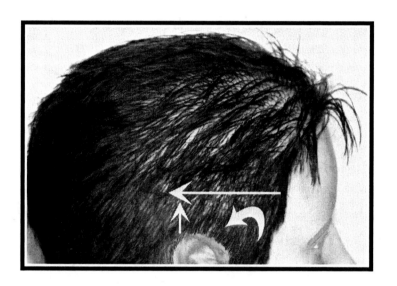

When both sides are complete, begin the back. Try not to clip any higher than the length of the sides using them as your guide. This will allow you to create a more balanced cut. Remember to slowly clip up and away from the head towards yourself to blend the two lengths together. (See figure 5 below.)

Figure #5

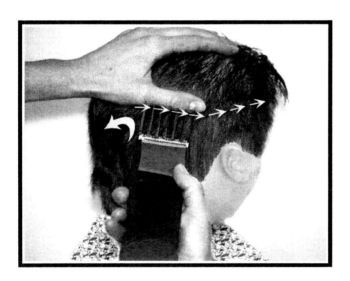

If you still want the sides shorter, continue with the next shortest guard. In this case, remove the guard that is now on your clipper, and replace it with the guard labeled ½ inch. This guard is still pretty easy to blend to the top, so continue to follow the same procedures on pages 106-108. (See figure 6 below.)

Figure #6

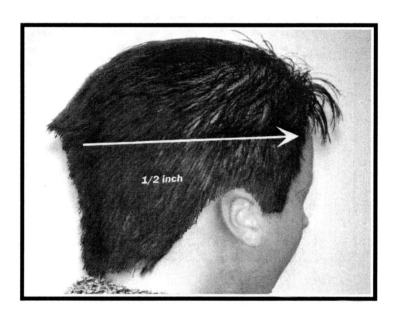

If you decide to go shorter than the ½ of an inch guard on the sides and back, follow these next few steps to gradually blend the hair:

First, replace the ½ inch guard with the 3/8 inch guard.

Continue to use your thumb as a guide, but place it just below the previous length that you clipped. Only clip up to your thumb. It will make it easier for you to blend. By blending the hair you will remove any harsh lines in the hair.

Remain consistent when placing your thumb just below the previous length, so the cut will become more balanced. (See figure 7 below.)

Figure #7

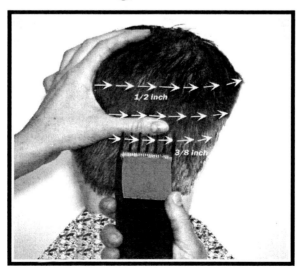

Complete the sides and back with the 3/8 inch guard. (See figure 8 below.)

Figure #8

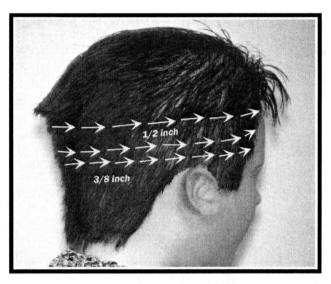

Follow the same procedures on the previous pages to go a little shorter. This time remove the 3/8 inch guard and replace it with the ¼ inch guard.

To go even shorter than ¼ of an inch, replace the ¼ inch guard with the 1/8 inch guard.

Begin with the sides. Place your thumb just below the length of the ¼ inch guard. Make sure that it stays in a consistent position throughout the cut.

When the sides are this short, it is easier to clipper the hair sideways rather than straight up. (See figure 9 below.)

Figure #9

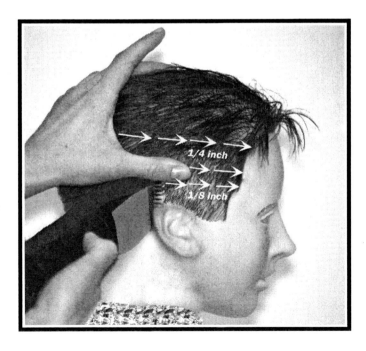

When you clip the back, remove the hair up and away from yourself slowly. (See figure 10 below.)

Figure #10

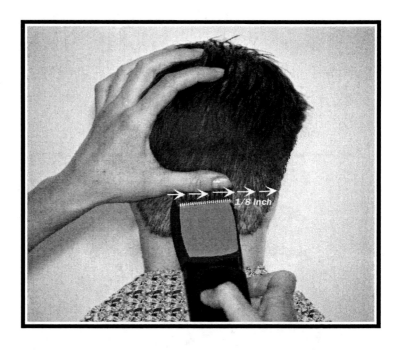

If you are satisfied with the length around the head, use your clippers to trim the sideburns to the desired length.

Carefully use the blade that is already attached, or the shortest blade that you have.

If you own a pair of trimmers, use them. (See figure 11 below.)

Figure #11

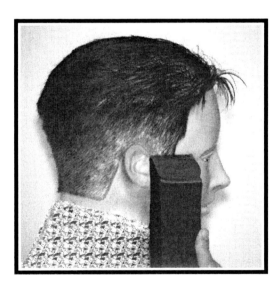

Now, clean up any unwanted hairs on the back of the neck.

Some people prefer a squared or rounded neckline. Define the neckline to the desired shape. (See figure 12 below.)

Figure #12

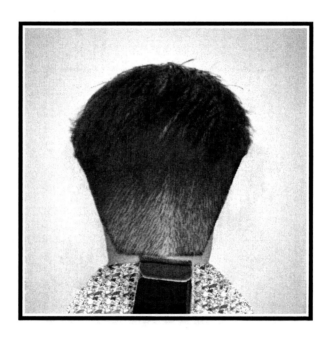

Look over the cut, and decide if it is short enough. If you want it shorter, simply go through each appropriate step starting on page 107. Going any shorter with your clippers will remove almost all of the hair. If you feel confident enough, you can use the already existing blade.

I do not recommend going this short until you are sure that you will be able to blend the hair.

If you do decide to go this short, start out by clipping the sides *a little* higher than just above the eyebrows so that you have enough room to go shorter. Use the same technique throughout this chapter and remember to take your time so that the hair blends correctly.

Finish the haircut by cleaning up the sideburns and the hair on the neck.

You now know how to complete a haircut using clippers!

Afterward

There are several different techniques to cut hair; but you must start with the basics.

Keep an open mind, think positive, learn all that you can, and have fun while you learn. Always take that opportunity to learn more. Once you find the most comfortable technique for yourself, master it!

After you complete the four haircuts in this book, you will become more familiar with the procedures. Eventually, you will not need to follow them systematically. You will be able to accomplish them on your own, or with very little guidance from this book.

For whatever reason you chose this book, I am glad that I could share my knowledge with you. I hope that it will help you to reach your goal whatever it may be.

Please feel free to share with me any comments or suggestions that you may have. We all learn from each other....

Lisa Marie Viggiano
P.O. Box 500868
Malabar, FL. 32950

TO PLACE AN ORDER:

Go to www. l-jpublishingandgraphics.com

Call 321-724-9004
OR
Send a check or money order to:
L&J Publishing and Graphics
P.O. Box 500868 Malabar, FL 32950

$17.95 per book

Quantity   *X*

RECEIVE FREE SHIPPING FOR A LIMITED
TIME ONLY AT:
www.l-jpublishingandgraphics.com

+.*06% sales tax for Fl residents only*

Total   = _____

*(Please include your name, address,
phone #, and book title)*